LIVING WITH CANCER

A Journey of Hope

*My personal story of the power
of positive thinking*

Margot Larson

My thanks to Sharon, Linda, Irene, Mary and Amber for their input, feedback and encouragement.

My gratitude to Don Ames for the cover photo and to Gardner Group Graphic Design LLC for cover design.

My heartfelt thanks to Dr. Scott Gettinger and Dr. Lynn Tanoue and the entire Thoracic Oncology team at Yale New Haven - Smilow Cancer Hospital for guiding my path on this journey.

Introduction

This book is not intended to present expert advice but rather practical, level-headed guidance for anyone whose life has been turned upside down by the prospect of cancer or other serious illness.

This helpful guide is written by a cancer patient, someone who has experienced the journey and who is recognized as someone who has a gift for putting things into perspective, and shifting chaos into manageable bites. This is such a serious topic that it can't possibly be presented without a touch of humor.

"My goal is to get this book in the hands of a patient and/or caregiver within days of a suspected diagnosis, because this is what I wish I had when first faced with these challenges."

Margot Larson

CHAPTER 1 – IMMEDIATE ACTION REQUIRED

First Sign of Trouble
Suspected Diagnosis
Confirmation of Diagnosis
The Beginning of the Waiting Game
Reaction to the Surprise – Holy Shit !
Telling Family and Friends
First Meeting with the Oncologist
Prognosis – Statistics
Testing and Preparing for Treatment
Beginning Treatment
Don't Go at it Alone. Recruit and Delegate - Share
Get the Skinny – Know What You are Facing – Get a
Handle on the Situation
Mind over Matter -Imagine the best outcome
Line up the Medical Team
Clear the Calendar and Adjust Your Priorities
Doctor's Visits and Tests
A Port to Weather the Storm
Wading Through Treatment
Appoint an Advocate

CHAPTER 2 - NEXT STEP

Side Effects – Life is all About Tradeoffs
Level with the Medical Team
Be Hopeful – It's a Good Strategy
Become a Writer -Keep a Journal
Bet on Yourself
Speak Up – You Are Still in Charge
Complimentary Therapies – At the Cancer Center of
Everywhere
Scope out the Minefield -Identify Obstacles
Surround yourself with cheerleaders

CHAPTER 3 – HANG IN THERE and BUILD CHARACTER

Cut Yourself Some Slack
Acquire an Attitude and Manage Your Thoughts
Practice Courage
Take it One Day at a Time
Be Grateful and Nurture Your Team
If You Get Knocked Down – Get Up Again
Ask and Accept with Grace
Emotional Roller Coaster
Alternatives to Isolation
Grieving is a Natural Reaction
Be Creative
Pace Yourself -Take a Break

CHAPTER 4 – FACING THE FUTURE

Envision and Design the Future
Count Your Blessings
It's Your Life – You Are Still in Charge
Revisit Your Priorities
Make your Bucket List
Acknowledge the Gifts

CHAPTER 5 – A SPECIAL WORD FOR FAMILY, FRIENDS and CAREGIVERS

What To Say
What Not To Say
What You Can Do
Caring for the Caregiver

CHAPTER 1

IMMEDIATE ACTION

First Sign of Trouble

My cough and shortness of breath continue despite
the daily use of Advair, so I ask my primary care
physician whether my symptoms could be related to
heart function. There was heart disease in both my
mother's and my father's sides of the family; and in
fact my father died at age 69 of congestive heart
failure. My doctor does not attribute my symptoms
to heart, so she schedules a CT scan for me, even
though I had two x-rays over the previous three
months with no concerns.

I go for the scan at 8 AM and by 9:30 my doctor's
office is on the phone asking me to come in later
that day. When I arrive for my 5:30 PM
appointment, she meets me at the door and guides
me to her office. I sensed right then and there that
there was a problem.

We discuss the findings of tumors on my lung and
agree to schedule an appointment with the Chief of
Cardiovascular Surgery at a renown teaching
hospital, one hour away. Passing on the local
hospitals will become one of the great decisions that
I will make on this journey.

Suspected Diagnosis

I waited two miserable weeks for my appointment
with the cardiovascular doctor. He recommended a
biopsy and confirmed 3 tumors in my right lung
covering all 3 lobes. He indicated that it was
inoperable and that he was 95% sure it was cancer.
Yikes. What a dose of reality!

Confirmation of the Diagnosis

A week later, when the doctor calls with the results
of the biopsy, I ask him to please tell me the good
news first before sharing the bad news. And he
does. The good news is that my left lung is healthy.
The bad news is that I have three sizeable tumors in
my right lung, clasped around my pulmonary artery.
I am being referred to a lung cancer oncologist.
That appointment is another two weeks away.

The Beginning of the Waiting Game

First, there is the two weeks of waiting once we saw
the scan. Then, after the suspected diagnosis and the
biopsy, I wait for the appointment with the
Oncologist. Those four weeks were brimming with
emotion and steaming with anxiety and probably
the worst part of my experience. This is where the
system breaks down.

The day I met with the Oncologist I also met with
the social worker, dedicated to patients with lung
cancer. That felt very late in the process. Where was

my lifeline in the first 30 days - before the cancer center support chimed in? Who was there to advise me not to browse the internet where I might find something that would scare me even more? Who was available to guide me and prepare me?

Today, I know I could have gone to one of the lung cancer organizations for a Phone Buddy, or to a chat room to ask some questions of other cancer patients who would have provided support and mentoring. Wouldn't it be nice if the moment an appointment is scheduled, a telephone support system is established with a patient, even if it is determined later that a cancer diagnosis is a false alarm?

Reaction to the Surprise. Holy Shit!

Denial is the first reaction for some of us. *"It's a mistake." "It's probably benign." " It's minor – let's get rid of it." "But I'm perfectly healthy." "How could it be this serious when I have no symptoms, not a clue?" " I'm not sick."*

This is our survival instinct kicking in - a perfectly natural instinct and reaction.

When I got the news, I put on a strong front at the doctor's office and then I cried for four days. After that, they kept me busy with tests and more tests and a biopsy. I have since learned that the tissues acquired during a biopsy are critical later to identify whether you have certain mutations which can qualify you for a clinical trial. It can gain you access to new treatments and discoveries.

Since I am medically ignorant, there were a lot of questions I could have asked. It was too rushed. It was a crisis! We were in shock and did not even know the questions.

For instance, while I had the presence of mind to insist on being under anesthesia for the Medianoscopy and the Bronchoscopy, it did not occur to me at the time how they would position my head and neck for the procedure. If I had known, I would have alerted them that I have arthritis in my neck and need support whenever I am lying down, whether it is sleeping, a massage, or even exercising. I have difficulty holding my neck up without some support.

Whatever position I was in during the procedure, my neck was in agony when I awoke. Nothing else mattered. The incision, the internal bruising was negligible compared to the pain in the back of my neck.

Telling Family and Friends

My first call was to my closest friends. I had to practice sharing the news. It was hard to do without breaking down in tears. This was a frightening time in my life. I did not know the degree of seriousness; I did not know how or where we were headed.

I had a good friend who was dealing with bowel cancer and so she was my first call for reinforcement. My sister-in-law and good friend, Monique, had died of breast cancer seven years earlier from a battle that lasted fifteen years. I did not come away from these experiences with a good opinion of chemo. My husband and I cried often during the period of August 10th (the CT scan) to September 11th (meeting with the oncologist). By nature, I am a person of action rather than emotion. Knowledge is power. If I know the plan, I can handle it. Limbo is disastrous to my psyche.

First Meeting with the Oncologist

I didn't realize that one could bring an entourage to this first appointment. I assumed I could bring only one person, and so I asked my best friend's husband to accompany me because he had successfully battled throat cancer several years earlier. That was a mistake. My husband should have been there to walk with me through the start of this journey.

The initial meeting with an oncologist is overwhelming. There is so much information to absorb and process, so many questions to ask, so much emotion flowing. It's really hard to take it all in. In my case, I had such limited knowledge of my physical body; I didn't really know exactly where my lungs were located. Through necessity, I have come a long way since then.
This meeting included both medical and radiation oncologists, along with a few fellows. This is a

teaching hospital which means, that in addition to leading-edge treatment, we also have an extended family of doctors who follow the case, for a while. (It's really a rotation system.) I decided it was a benefit rather than an irritation or invasion of privacy. These medical students are the potential of future discoveries. I could either fight it or be part of the solution. I chose the latter.

Prognosis – Statistics

Some oncologists will candidly offer you their perception of the impact on your life expectancy. Others will ask whether you want to hear the prognosis, the life expectancy statistics.

This is an area of debate among cancer patients. Some are told early on that they have only 2-4 months to live. Six years later, they may still be alive yet traumatized by that original prediction. There are statistics gathered by cancer organizations that may apply to your situation. Yet, it is best to get that information from your oncologist; don't go looking for this on the internet. You could scare yourself to death or go into depression as a result of some inaccurate information.

Understand that every case is different, because we each enter our cancer journey with a different health status and different mental perspective. We each react to treatment differently. And most important, the treatment for cancer is changing so rapidly; targeted treatments sometimes may now be a first line of treatment. A few years ago, you could not participate in clinical trials unless you had tried all conventional treatments first. There have been so many improvements and new options since 2010 that I seriously question whether the statistics are current and applicable.

When asked about hearing the prognosis, I told my doctor that I did not want to hear the statistics, that I would rather write my own outcome. I have, since that time, accidentally come across some numbers on the internet and am happy that I did not hear them upon diagnosis. That information would have surely impaired my fighting spirit.

So I suggest you really think about what you want to know about timeframe, and tell your doctor upfront. The statistics assume that 50% of people will do better and 50% will do worse than the predictions. By the way, I already beat the statistics five years into my battle.

Testing and Preparing for Treatment

This phase requires a lot of tolerance. There are EKGs, Echo Cardiograms, CT Scans, MRIs, Pet Scans, perhaps X-Rays and ultrasounds, and few more I have not listed. Then in preparation for radiation, there is measuring, marking, testing, making a frame, whatever is needed to ensure right-on-target radiation.

Beginning Treatment

Probably the most daunting aspect is our nervousness over not knowing what will happen, how we are going to react (not to mention the buildup of our emotional state over the past few weeks). There is a lot of waiting that goes along with cancer treatment. The order for the chemo is usually given once you arrive at the cancer center. The cocktail gets mixed up to your specifications. And, there are many people arriving at the same time for treatment. Then there is waiting for approval from the doctor, who may be with another very sick patient or responding to an emergency. Come prepared to spend many hours. Bring a book, a laptop, needlepoint or whatever can occupy your mind during the treatment and the waiting. Bring some snacks that you like. Most cancer centers will feed you, but it's nice to enjoy your favorite things.

It's time to try to calm your body and your mind. Convince yourself that this is the right path, that it is a means to an end, that it will work and keep your stress level as low as possible. It is my experience, that the greeters, nurses, the volunteers, and the doctors are some of the most patient, warm, and compassionate people in my life. They do their best to treat me as an individual and make me feel that I am the most important person at that moment in time. It's time to go with the flow on one hand, and stay alert, interested and participate in managing your own treatment on the other hand. Ask questions. Explore. Learn. Your life is worth it. Keep notes of your body's reaction to everything.

During treatment, you can request to speak to a social worker or a chaplain if you wish. I was offered a massage in a private room where I went with my IV bag. Aside from your chemo cocktail, you will probably receive anti-nausea medication, hydration, and perhaps a steroid to help counter the impact.

How you will personally react to the chemo, or anything else you receive, can vary a great deal from others, and from one cycle to another. Read about the possible, probable and unusual reactions so you can recognize them.

Don't Go at it Alone. Recruit, Delegate, Share

You will encounter many, many reasons why you must reach out and call in favors and get help. Believe me when I say that your family and friends will feel privileged to be included and asked for help. (*More about this in Chapters 3 and 5.*) Don't shut people out. There is nothing to be embarrassed or ashamed of. Sharing will help you get to reality faster. This is not a time to hibernate or stick your head in the sand. There is a time to grieve your loss. (*See more about this Chapter 3.*)

Talking about cancer and your illness is emotional. You feel vulnerable. You lose control on one hand

and want re-assurance on the other. You are trying to project the seriousness, not the alarm.

Not Telling Someone can be Hurtful.

I tried to spare one of my friends, because she had been the caregiver for her childhood friend who had lost her battle with cancer the previous year. My friend's husband also died of cancer a few years earlier. In my desire to protect her from one more encounter with cancer, I realized later that I was unconsciously implying that she was not an intimate enough friend for me to share this experience with her. This is an example where intention and impact conflict.

Perhaps, it is not up to us to decide whether someone can handle it or not. Give them the chance to deal with the news, the information. Some people respond immediately. Others need to process. Don't judge. You have more important things to worry about.

Reach out for help. Call in the troops. If not now, when? Isn't this one of the most important moments of your life? Cash in those chips you've accumulated. While some of us want to be the givers, the rescuers - we must however also learn to receive and accept.

I identified what I considered to be my inner circle. I sent a note to those people and told them so, giving them permission to call me, to ask whatever questions they had and I asked them to communicate outwardly and to protect me from what could be time and energy consuming communications from the outer circle. I created a site on caringbridge.org where I posted regular updates. My friends, family and business colleagues still appreciate it today because it keeps them posted without having to call us and disturb us during this crisis. You can also have a friend send regular updates to a mailing list you create.

Get the Skinny – Know What You are Facing – Get a Handle on the Situation

This is not a time to let your imagination run wild. Get a medical perspective. Ask about the options. Talk to others who have faced a similar situation. Ask for referrals. Check out the biographies of your medical staff and institutions. Do not rely on your family doctor as your point of cancer care. Find a recommended oncologist who specializes in your type of cancer.

Ask where your primary cancer is located and whether there is metastasis to other locations. Ask about the type of cancer and the stage. All of this may be meaningless to you at this point, but will be important as you digest the information and are faced with decisions about your treatment. Write it down for the future. It's a great idea to take someone with you to take notes. You can even think through some questions with them beforehand. Make them your personal secretary to support you. I have done this many times. And if you don't remember something when you get home, call the doctor and ask again. They understand that you are not capable of absorbing a lot of information at one time.

Keep in mind there may be better institutions out-of-state, and weigh the pros and cons of selecting an out-of-state facility. I chose Yale's Smilow Cancer Hospital, located one hour from my home - not the closest hospital, but close enough. I personally could not imagine having to commute to New York City or temporarily reside in Texas during my treatment. It would be another loss to:

- Not be able to cuddle up by the fireplace or enjoy my own comfortable bed.
- Have to live in a hotel room in between treatments.
- Not have access to our neighbors/friends who became an invaluable support to us.

However, if I did not have an outstanding cancer center in my state, or had not connected with the right physicians, I would have done whatever it took to get the best care. It's about survival and making the best choices.

Mind over Matter: Imagine the Best Outcome

This is critical to recovery. Do whatever it takes to get to a place of optimism and positive mindset.

Before I underwent a protocol of very aggressive chemotherapy and radiation, I had to retreat for a few days to shift my beliefs. Until then, I had never believed in chemo. I viewed it as an evil, a poison as lethal as cancer. I had to believe that taking this poison would in fact cure me.

I encourage you to approach your therapy in the same way. You must believe that it will work. There is no room for doubt. You must imagine the best possible outcome and believe it.

It is difficult to go about your life and not have cancer or the fear overwhelm your every moment. It's like a dark cloud following you around. Wendy Levin Peterson, APRN, at Middlesex Hospital Cancer Center, suggests to her patients that they create a cancer box in their head. This may help you keep the lid on the chaos by compartmentalizing it. Close your eyes and see your box. Open it up only when you need to deal with it.

What I have learned, down the road, is the ability to get beyond the fear and the anxiety to a point that you focus on the present and find ways to minimize stress in your life. I consider this to be the ultimate success of this journey.

Line Up the Medical Team

In *Cancer Today*, Hester Hill Schnipper, Chief of Oncology social work at Beth Israel Deaconess

Medical Center in Boston, reminds us
"Relationships go both ways and it is safe to assume
that your doctor wants good communication with
you."

I got lucky! When I discussed the options with my
primary care physician, we passed on local hospitals
and I opted for a referral to a teaching hospital.
Somehow I started with the Chief of Cardiovascular
Surgery and continued with referrals to the most
talented of physicians and medical providers.
Second opinions are important and actually critical
if your first stop implies limited hope. Find out how
your medical team works within their organization.

Hester Hill Schnipper also suggests that you tell
your doctor a little about yourself. Force some
normal social interaction. Having information
about your life will help your doctor relate to you as
a real person.

My medical team participates in a weekly Tumor
Board where cases are discussed and there is the
opportunity for other opinions and approaches.
That was reassuring to me.
My medical oncologist regularly confers with others
to review reports.

I think it is important for you to like, respect, and
trust your doctor, to feel confident and comfortable
with him or her. If the connection isn't there, move
on to another. There are plenty of talented medical
professionals. Don't worry about hurting their

feelings. Keep it in perspective. This is no time to be "wimpy" when the rest of your life is at stake.

Ask, so you know with certainty, "Who's on first?" Who is in charge? This becomes critical when you deal with many physicians.

If you are being treated for lung cancer, and you become congested because of spring allergies, or you have difficulty sleeping, do you go to your primary physician, the pulmonologist or your medical oncologist? Know this information before you need it. Schnipper also suggests, "Ask how to reach your doctor between appointments. Are emails OK? Will your doctor or a nurse return the call? Don't call with minor questions that can wait."

You may want to seek out a counselor to help you and/or your spouse and children along this difficult journey. Utilize the services of the social worker assigned to your cancer department, the chaplain at the cancer center or your pastor. Your life has changed in an instant, and you are going to need all the help you can get to get through and beyond this challenge.

Clear the Calendar and Adjust your Priorities

Career, work, family should no longer come first. It's about **you** and your health.
If you do not address this as your top (and only) priority, you may not be around to take care of the

rest. In everything you do, your schedule, your promises, ask yourself, "Is this in the best interest of my recovery? In the scope of life, how important is this?"

It is amazing how tolerant we become once we have been challenged with adversity. The petty things don't rattle me anymore.

- So what if I have to wait one hour to see my doctor?
- So what if someone flips me off while driving on the highway?
- So what if someone cuts in front of me in line?

It may not be nice. It may not be right. And it just isn't that important anymore.
There is a certain amount of freedom that comes when facing your mortality.

Since stress contributes to disease, I take great pleasure in eliminating stressful situations in my life. I have opted not to continue serving certain customers who are "high maintenance" and cause me stress. I avoid people who are whiners, who see only the negatives or who smoke. I will pay more for a non-stop flight, because I dislike takeoffs and landings and prefer to minimize them. These are just a few of the stressful situations I choose not to include in my life.

Doctor's Visits and Tests

- Prepare for your visit with the doctor. Make a list of questions.
- Keep a log of your symptoms and concerns.
- Maintain an appointment/treatment calendar.
- Provide test schedulers with your input as to when it is most convenient for you.

Sometimes you just can't wait for the scheduled appointment to ask a question because it is urgent or impacts other decisions. It's OK for you to call your doctor, leave a message, and ask for a call back. Remember: They work for you.
I always feel it is best when leaving a message to pose my question or tell them why I am calling. It may expedite a return call. You don't want to abuse this process, nor do you want to shy away from it.

- I find my doctor's nurse practitioner to be very helpful. She is almost always able to answer my questions, prescribe medication, recommend and approve a test, or ask the doctor to call me. She is highly responsive. Some cancer centers have a "nurse navigator." Ask whether there is such a person on your team.

- For most people, it's a good idea to take someone with you to appointments. It's a back up. They will hear what you may not. They can help pose questions you might forget. They are calmer and probably more objective.

- When your doctor recommends certain tests and suggests certain medication, remember to get the prescriptions before you leave the office.

- I prefer to schedule the tests myself so that I can coordinate the time and place with my schedule or preferred driving time. Occasionally, when I call to schedule a test I am told they do not yet have the order from the doctor. I just call back later.

Prescriptions: Remember that the doctor's office must either call it in or fax it to the pharmacy. Your other choice is to get a signed script to present to the pharmacy.

What does not work: The pharmacy will not accept a photocopy or a prescription fax from the patient. Keep in mind that some pharmacies do not carry certain narcotics and you may have to go to an out-of-town pharmacy. This is an excellent time to ask a friend or neighbor for help in picking up that prescription for you.

A word of caution: do not wait until you run out to call for a refill or ask the doctor for a new prescription. There can be a delay of several days at the doctor's office as well as a wait for authorization from the insurance company.

As you progress in your care, you will be told that the doctor wants to see you in two months and/or you need a CT scan or other test in three months. Schedule it **now** while it's clear in your mind and mark your calendar immediately. It's always easier to schedule way in advance and reschedule, if you have to, rather than wait and not be able to get the date you want.

If you are scheduling a CT scan or similar test to see whether your cancer has progressed, retreated or returned, schedule that test no more than 2-3 days before your doctor's appointment. The period of time between the test and the doctor's visit is usually a time of high anxiety – no matter how often or how long you have been doing this.

I always request a copy of my blood work report and my diagnostic tests so I can review, compare them and prepare additional questions. I obtain a CD of my scans and carry my medical journal with me whenever I travel for more than a couple of days. It has been helpful when I have landed in an emergency center.

Emergencies: If you require immediate medical care, start with your cancer center and whomever is on call. If you go to a hospital emergency room, ask them to communicate with your oncologist immediately before starting care or treatment. Be careful not to let them treat you for the symptoms they are observing and overlook the primary and most important problem: cancer.

Some of the test reports appear to be written in a foreign language. You will probably need your doctor to interpret them. I sometimes take the time to check out some of the terminology in a dictionary or Wikipedia to understand the terms. Don't be shy about asking someone to review your X-Ray or Scan and show you the areas of concern. It's their job to educate you about your condition.

A Port to Weather the Storm

An oncology nurse advised that anyone with advanced cancer is going to be in treatment or need labs/scans frequently, and probably the remainder of their life, and a port will prove to be a blessing. Insist it be a power port so it can also be used to infuse contrast dye. Here are the differences:

- **An IV** is a needle in your arm to enable infusions and to draw blood. Often when you've had chemo infusions, it affects your veins and nurses may not get a good vein on a first try. If you are hospitalized, they draw blood at least once a day so that's a lot of needle sticks.

- **A pic line** is like an IV but it's done once. The line is installed and stays in and allows ongoing access. It is temporary but it really helps reduce the needle sticks.

- **A port** is installed surgically in your chest or arm. It's not visible unless you are looking for it. It can be accessed as needed and the needle can stay in for daily need. Generally access is not painful. If the needle is replaced weekly or more frequently the area will be sensitive. If this is the case, it is recommended that you use EMLA cream an hour before accessing the port in order to numb the area. I found that removing the needle was painless and actually my husband was taught to remove it so I could have a good shower before the next round. It is important to keep the area sterile to prevent infection.

There are variations of ports, in size and for different uses. A power port allows the use of the port to insert the dye for contrast which goes in a high rate of speed, as opposed to chemo, antibiotics, or hydration, which go in slowly.

Wading Through Treatment

<u>Radiation</u>

The actual process of radiation seems easy compared to chemo, at least that was my experience with lung cancer. Obviously, it can be far more invasive and uncomfortable for other types of cancer. There are no needles, no chemicals, no immediate effects. Once the preparation is over, it usually takes more time to get undressed for it than to actually get it.

The side effects usually show up after a few weeks. Fatigue is one of them and it can be pretty overwhelming when Radiation is done simultaneously with chemo treatment. Skin burns are also another side effect. In the case of lung or other chest area treatments, the burns were worse on my back than on my chest. My husband treated the burns with pads soaked with saline in order to remove the heat, and then we used cream.

The other side effect was that, along with zapping the lung tumors, areas close to the targeted area also get burned. In my case it was the esophagus. It was so irritated or inflamed that I had difficulty eating. So ironically, at a time when I needed nutrients the most, my body wanted to reject foods and liquids. I lost weight quickly, but I don't recommend it as a diet plan!

Infusions

Chemo infusions are delivered in cycles and everyone's individual treatment plan varies. You might get chemo a couple of days a week; the cycle might run 1-3 weeks with a break of a few weeks before you start the next cycle.
The cumulative effect of the infusions will impact some patients sooner than others. Some get several different drugs as part of their cycle, others just one. The amount of the dosage will have an impact, and your condition prior to starting treatment will also play a role in how you will react.

It is advisable that you get a ride to treatment, because you don't know how you will react and how tired or weak you may be after treatment. In addition to the chemo, you may get infusions of supportive meds to counter the impact of certain drugs. Hydration is often part of the treatment as are some steroids.

You may want to give thought to the time of the day that you agree to schedule your treatment. Consider the length of your commute, traffic volume for your commute back and forth, the time of the day that you feel your best, when you can get a ride, and how long you can expect to be there. Always assume that you will be there twice as long as they tell you the treatment should last.

If you do not have a dedicated caregiver, this is the time for you to start a list of potential rides from all those people who have offered to help, and assign days. Keep a list of your reactions so you can accurately report them to your oncology team. If they know how you are responding, they can provide counter measures such as a B-12 shot, or other booster, perhaps increase hydration, monitor your vitals more closely, adjust your dosage, give you something to sleep or to minimize your anxiety.

While it is a good time in your life to review your nutrition, and make adjustments, you may find that during treatment the loss of appetite, the metallic taste in your mouth or your body's elimination system may cause you to avoid certain foods. You may need to eat anything that appeals to you in order to get nutrients and/or proteins.

One of my friends delivered all kinds of good foods from the health food store helping me to change my diet in accordance with the many books that tell us what we should or should not eat. I agree that though it may be time for a lifestyle review and adjustment, your body is already under a great deal of stress, so you need to identify the foods that will be both healthy and consumable for you at this time in your treatment.

No one told me not to have liquor or wine during treatment, or to stop having my nails done or my hair died. These were things that I stopped because it made good sense to me. My energy would be drained further if I had a cocktail. I chose to avoid fumes and chemicals that might interact with the drugs now entering my body. Remember that some of this is temporary and so you should feel comfortable tweaking and adjusting as you progress through treatment.

During treatment, it is important that you listen to your body and rest. You need to pamper yourself. You may want to keep your mind challenged, though some of us actually find it difficult focusing and reading. I found audio books and movies are good entertainment.

I have met individuals who continued to work full time through their treatment and/or maintain a disciplined exercise routine. I applaud them though I did not emulate them. My advice on this topic is to think through and clarify your priorities. What is

most important at this point of your life? In my
case, it was anything I could do to regain health and
be well. Make conscious decisions.
Today, clinical trials are often available as a first
line of treatment. Just a few years ago, those trials
were only available when the conventional
treatment was not working for the patient. Many
clinical trials are oral medication which can result in
a broad spectrum of side effects that will vary
depending on the dosage, the drug, and how long
you've been on it.

Today, treatment for some cancers are targeted to
your particular cancers, DNA, mutations, etc. They
have identified drugs that work specifically for us,
as individuals. That's why we often repeat biopsies
as they identify more details about your specific
cancer cells. I remember my oncologist telling me
that they had tested the tissue of 300 patients, and I
was the only match of this new drug that was
coming to clinical trial.

I usually search for a discussion with people with
similar cancer and perhaps taking the same drug.
The exchange of information is good for all
concerned. The newly diagnosed learn from the
experience of others; those who have travelled the
path can pay it forward and be of great help to
others. The internet is good for connecting with
others, learning how they have coped and to gain
hope. The internet is not the place to view
prognosis, statistics, or to scare you to an early
death by reading inaccurate information from a non-

professional site. If you are researching, go to the national cancer organizations and reputable cancer centers.

When I was researching pleural effusion, I came across a comment from someone who claimed that if you have pleural effusion you are usually dead within six months. That was a non-educated opinion and it was scary to read as I had a pleural drain for 5 months. That was several years ago, I'm still here years later and actually doing quite well.

Appoint an Advocate

This is very important. There will be times when you are not up to hearing all the data that is being sent your way. I have had several instances walking out of the doctor's office believing I heard the doctor say one thing, and my husband recounted the exact opposite. When I checked with the doctor, my husband was right. This was a mind blower for me because I fully believed that my mind was clear and objective. In fact, we may hear very little of what the doctor says. So be prepared.

Take someone along with you, to hear, to record, and to repeat to you. They can ask the questions you might want to ask but are not able or comfortable asking. If you don't have someone to go with you to an appointment, reschedule the appointment. Aside from my husband, I have taken along an oncology nurse friend, someone with EMT training, a cancer patient and close friends who are detail-oriented and would have my best interest at heart. Whomever you choose must be objective, willing and able to understand, know and support your choices and beliefs. (Your other option is to tape the conversation, which will help confirm later what the doctor said.)

Several states have healthcare advocacy offices/units which are a great resource, should there be any problem with insurance companies denying treatment. Calling sooner rather than later is important, as they will walk you through the appeal process, even attend an appeals hearing with you or your caregiver or appointee, if need be. My state has an exceptionally high success rate in overturning denials. Check whether you have the same resource in your state. There are also some non-profit and community healthcare advocacy programs available.

Another option is hiring a healthcare advocate consultant which I have done on two occasions. The savings they negotiated on my behalf was significantly more than their consultant fee. I have also utilized this service to help me select my Medicare supplements and review other insurance options.

CHAPTER 2

NEXT STEP

Side Effects – Life is All about Trade-Offs

Your doctor or cancer center will provide you with information describing the chemotherapy drug(s) or other treatment and what the side effects are. I noticed that some of this is limited and represents only the most common side effects. I found it helpful to supplement my knowledge by going to the drug company's site and read more about the drug's track record and its side effects. Don't panic at some of the side effects that occur in rare cases. The purpose is to be aware and informed, because we all react differently.

A word of caution: be skeptical about the sources of information on the internet. Don't believe everything you read. Stick to bona-fide cancer center and hospital websites and recognized national cancer organizations.

Another source of learning about side effects is talking with other patients who have used that particular drug. Remember that treatments affect everyone differently. Our bodies are in varying states of health and different levels of disease. Our sensitivities and reactions vary. The reason I wanted to know about the side effects, in advance, is simply to recognize them if they do occur.

Bone or Muscle Damage –In my case, it wasn't until one year after my initial treatment that I learned that a potential side effect of my chemo was weakening of the bones and muscles. This along with the steroids I was taking resulted in Avascular Necrosis, destroying my hip joint and requiring a total hip replacement.

Your Looks - I was so determined to not look sick that I made every effort to always look good. I opted to use makeup, to wear colorful and flattering clothes and a wig that fooled almost everyone. There are resources to help you with your image. Some cancer centers provide free wigs and scarves. The American Cancer Society offers free wigs and conducts monthly "Look Good - Feel Better" programs at most cancer centers. Ask the social worker at your cancer center about such resources. In my case, whenever I feel that I look good, it definitely helps me feel better about myself.

Hair Loss –For me, this was the most devastating side effect of chemotherapy. My beautiful long blond hair fell out two weeks after the start of my chemo and did so in a period of 12 hours. I never had a chance to get used to the idea. And then for weeks afterwards, I found hair all over my house, my bed, my car. Ask your doctor whether this can be a side effect of your chemo. I was told that it would be, but I thought I could will my way around it.

What I would do differently: As soon as I was told that my hair would probably fall out, I would immediately have my hair cut into a very short hairstyle and then buy a matching wig. That way, when my hair did fall out, the transition would be seamless, though perhaps still painful (literally and figuratively). You may be surprised to learn that your entire scalp becomes very sensitive, as hair falls out, just as if someone was actually pulling it out. You may lose hair elsewhere including your eyebrows. A friend found eyebrow stencils and powder at the local pharmacy that worked very well.

I resented anyone telling me, "Don't let it bother you, it will grow back. It is not a big deal. Don't worry about it." It is a big deal! I felt a loss of my identity. There was a stranger staring me in the mirror. I felt naked.

Nausea – I recall little or no problem with nausea with my chemo infusions, and that may be uncommon. You will usually be given anti-nausea medication along with your chemo. It is important for you to assume you will have nausea, have the medication on hand and take it before you begin vomiting. That's why it is given to you. Think about it. If you wait until you begin to vomit, you won't be able to keep down the medication. You want to prevent the problem before it occurs. It's no different than with pain medication. If you wait until the pain is unbearable to take your pain meds, then it may take a long time for the meds to take effect and the pain to subside. Take the meds before the situation gets out of hand.

It may be a good idea to ask your doctor for a prescription for suppositories for nausea so you can have it on hand in the event you can't keep anything down, and therefore can't take the medication by mouth. The oral chemo (clinical trial) I began taking in 2010 caused serious nausea and I dared not consume it before taking anti-nausea medication. I have had a violent response when taking these meds on an empty stomach.

Constipation and Diarrhea – These are both common side effects and you may get one or the other. So, depending on your reaction, you can use nutrition as a way to help control and counter the effect. If you are constipated, increase your fiber. If you have diarrhea, watch out for caffeine and other diuretics. Follow the standard advice for these conditions.

Radiation Burns -Another difficult side effect that was a result of my radiation were significant burns on my chest, and even more seriously on my back, which required daily treatment. Thank God my husband was capable and willing to doctor me. In addition, my esophagus was so badly irritated and burned from radiation. I seemed unable to swallow food. And just how much vanilla pudding, milkshakes, and nutritional drinks can you consume? It was easier not to eat. And yet, intellectually I understood my husband's fear and frustration that if I did not get enough nutrients, I would be unable to fight back, to sustain the treatment and begin healing. When I attempted to shove the food and liquids down, my "gag factor" would act up. I lost 25 lbs in 3 weeks (from a size 12 to a size 6). By the way, this is why doctors tell you to "bulk up" before starting treatment and to continue to consume whatever food appeals to you during treatment. Your body needs strength and stamina to survive and thrive.

It helps you to 'know your body" and it requires that you pay attention to the signals your body sends you. You must keep monitoring the changes and rely on a close friend or family member to do the same, just in case you become lackadaisical about it.

Fatigue is a common side effect. Your body needs strength to absorb the treatment and fight the disease. You can't afford to do anything that will interfere or reduce your energy level. This type of fatigue is not eliminated through sleep. You may get up in the morning, after eight hours of sleep, and feel just as tired as when you went to bed. I remember sitting on the sofa and having the thought that I needed a glass of water or to go to the bathroom, and it would take me 20 minutes to act on that thought. Keep in mind that it is temporary.

During (and for a long period after) treatment, alcoholic cocktails were out of the question for me. They robbed energy. So does stress. So does lack of sleep. I began to take naps for the first time in my life.

Sleepiness and/or Insomnia
I often found myself sleeping nine to eleven hours per night, even long after chemo treatment was over. My body needed it. Sometimes, it was simply that I did not have the energy to get up in the morning when I woke up. And that's OK.

On the other end of the spectrum, some patients will be unable to fall asleep or stay asleep. Some of this may be the result of steroids administered along with your chemo or a reaction to your particular chemo drug. Look for ways to at least rest, if you can't sleep. Recommendations to help you get to sleep include: deep breathing, meditation, imagery, warm milk, and certain foods such as bananas, reading, or taking a warm bath. Doctors usually advise against getting up and doing housework, un-cluttering your home office, or playing on the internet. As a matter of fact, I have read many articles cautioning us about the effect of computer use or stimulating activity just before bedtime. I also found it helpful not to look at the clock, to avoid convincing myself that I would be exhausted in the morning, since I was still awake at 2 AM.

Anxiety and Depression

Along with fatigue and low energy, often come discouragement, anxiety, and a rollercoaster of emotions as we face a serious illness. This can occur at any point in time: during initial testing, at diagnosis stage, during cancer treatment, and even upon completion of cancer treatment. It is important to let your healthcare team know if you are experiencing emotional, psychological, or spiritual distress.

Most cancer centers provide a range of psychological health services. If available, consider starting with an oncology social worker. They are trained to help you and your family deal with a range of psychosocial issues through counseling to address your fears and concerns, as well as provide referral to hospital-based or community resources.

Some patients benefit from individual therapy and/or medications such as antidepressants. If psychotropic medication is suggested, evaluation by a psychiatrist or psychiatric nurse practitioner will be offered. Some centers have psychologists who may assist with counseling around emotional and psychological difficulties, but who cannot prescribe medication. You may want to check with your insurance company for a list of preferred mental health providers, as well as the coverage for the cost of this service.

Many patients experience spiritual and existential concerns when faced with a potentially life-threatening illness. Some patients utilize complementary therapies for stress management such as yoga, guided imagery, Reiki, and massage.

Another resource for patients and families is to participate in a cancer support group or a peer support program. Many such groups are available at local hospitals and cancer centers as well as a variety of online chat groups, often narrowed to your specific cancer and medication. There is a great deal of information that you can learn from other patients who have travelled a similar journey. The following are additional organizations that may be able to direct you to support resources in your area:

Cancer Support Community	888-793-9855
CancerCare	800-813-HOPE (4673)
American Cancer Society	800-227-2345
Lung Cancer Alliance.org	800-298-2436

Hydration

No matter what your side effects are, you will realize that drinking plenty of water is critical to the process. You want to detox your system which means "what goes in must come out". You may find yourself measuring both intake and output. I have learned that it is critical during and after cancer treatment to ensure that your liver and gallbladder are operating at optimum efficiency. You can request a liver function test from your oncologist. I learned that acupuncture can help with liver function, as well as some of the other side effects of treatment, such as nausea, insomnia, etc.

Level With the Medical Team

It's beneficial to become very aware of your body and its reactions, so you can differentiate between what is a minor change and what feels odd. Be honest and tell the oncologists and team members the truth and what exactly is happening.

Early on, in my effort to be continuously positive and optimistic, I would always say I was doing fine. One day my husband told the doctor, "she lies a lot." I suddenly realized how foolish I was. I needed to report honestly so they could take action and protect me from serious consequences.

Generally, I have looked healthier than I am at any given time. That can be misleading. Last year, when I noticed that there was something very wrong, it took awhile to get everyone's attention. I had to really speak up and tell them that I felt really bad, the worst I had ever felt, and that I was spiraling down. It was finally determined that I had contracted an unusual infection in my bad lung, an infection that could require a high dose of antibiotics daily for more than a year; an infection that could have killed me.

The goal is to become aware and knowledgeable without being paranoid or alarmist.

Tell your doctor what you are worried and scared about. Be specific. Are you concerned about pain? Medical expenses? Caring for your children? Being a burden to your family? Your doctor or his/her support team may be able to guide you and refer you to resources that can provide you with some peace of mind.

Be Hopeful – It's a Good Strategy

I can tell you categorically that if I had known the survival statistics at the beginning, it would have impaired my spirit, positivity and determination. Being hopeful has its benefits. If you think you can beat it, your chances are much better. The best remedy to beat serious illness is hope. Don't misplace it. I suggest you do not go looking for those survival statistics, cure statistics, incidence of recurrence, etc. If you accidentally come across them, remember that they are "mean numbers" which means that 50% of people do better and 50% do worse.

When I first faced cancer, I was determined to be a "trooper." I recall asking my oncologists, "What percent of your patients don't have any side effects?" They responded 10%, and I told them I planned to be in that group.
Actually, I did do very well and still claim to have had little or no side effects. However, it's quite possible that my optimism short circuits my memory. Just like a woman giving birth, if we clearly remembered the discomfort and pain of birthing, we might not do it again, so our brain helps us misplace that memory.

Some may think that being hopeful will lead to disappointment. That's a possibility. However, I have observed that a hopeful spirit is happier, more successful, and more pleasant to be around than someone who always expects and imagines the worst. In the end, it's your choice, whether you want to focus on the glass half full or half empty.

Become a Writer -Keep a Journal

I always prided myself on having an excellent memory, but somehow this experience has impacted that. Some refer to it as "chemo brain", others as age. I think it is brain shock combined with overload. Whatever the cause, keep a journal of how you feel, track the changes, the side effects you experience; keep your list of medications, dates of appointments and CT scans. Maintain a list of questions you have for the doctor. My medical journal accompanies me to appointments and travels with me whenever I go out of state.

A second journal (or diary) should record your feelings, your fears, and observations. Use it to express yourself. Don't keep it all in. Keep a log like an old sea captain, an explorer, or a teenager. I have realized that I now need to keep a log on the refrigerator door of when I take my meds, otherwise I can't remember whether I took it an hour ago, or if I was just thinking about taking it.

A friend related keeping a "Friggit List" on which she listed insurance companies who deny coverage and anyone or anything that caused her stress and made her life more difficult on this journey. It's a good way to get it out of your system - acknowledge it and move beyond it. Do not let anger and frustration consume you. You have far greater hurdles to jump.

Bet on Yourself

Challenge the odds. Believe in the possibilities. Look for small successes so far. In some ways, you may be lucky. Find those nuggets and hang on to them. You must act successful before you become successful. If you think you can do it, you probably can. If you think you can't do it, you won't.

There are plenty of stories of cancer patients who were given 2-4 months to live and six or twelve years later, they are still around. A doctor's best guess can be wrong. There is no expiration date on the soles of our feet. Our approach to cancer and our body's ability to fight can outsmart the prediction.

Speak Up – You Are Still in Charge

You have to know enough to ask the right questions. You need to know your rights.
You want to partner with the medical staff and you want to push back when appropriate.

One of the directives I got when undergoing chemo was that if my temperature rose to 100.5, I had to seek urgent care. So one evening when my temperature hit 101, I called the cancer center. My doctor was not on call. The physician on call did not have access to my file, and so he insisted I go to an emergency center. I really wanted him to say, "Take two aspirins and call me in the morning." – But no such luck.

I went to the closest emergency room, which was dirty, full of people with colds and flu, a place I should not have been exposed to with a compromised immune system. The intake nurse suspected a 24-hour bug that was going around. I went through the system and the doctor I saw felt I had pneumonia and wanted to begin intravenous antibiotics immediately.

When I asked whether the antibiotic would interfere with my chemo treatment, he indicated that it might. I told him that I did not want the antibiotics until we could reach my oncologist. It was now 10 PM. The ER doctor was not pleased by my refusing to accept his recommendation, and I had to sign myself out "against medical advice." I tried to explain to him that we were dealing with life and death. The pneumonia would not kill me within the next 24 hours, but discontinuing chemo could affect my life. His focus was on the immediate situation rather than the big picture. He was treating only the condition that brought me to the emergency room.

The lesson I learned is that if you must go to an emergency room, always be sure that you ask them to contact a member of your oncology team <u>before</u> beginning treatment. They should never be treating the condition that brings you to this urgent care facility without having access to your case file. It turned out that when my oncology team saw the x-ray taken in the ER, they did not agree that I had, and they also informed me that antibiotics would not interfere would my chemo.

Another example is that of Brad, who required a bone marrow transplant for his Hodgkin's disease in 2003. His local cancer center on the east coast went ahead and scheduled this procedure, but Brad realized that they performed very few transplants and that he had to take control of his treatment. He refused to go ahead with the scheduled treatment.

He researched and found the top 10 cancer centers with significant bone marrow transplant experience, visited some and then opted to move temporarily to the west coast for treatment at the Fred Hutchinson Cancer Center in Seattle, where more than 250 transplants are performed every year.

Brad was an avid sailor and boating enthusiast who refused to let his transplant keep him away from a boat. In between his first few doctor's appointments, Brad immediately set about finding a way to get out on the beautiful Seattle waters.

Staff workers at the medical center told him about The Mallory Todd, a boat that took cancer patients out on day trips and sunset boat rides. Brad became a frequent passenger and volunteer over his four-month stay in Seattle.

Brad's sister Melissa, founded R.A.C.E. (Remission and Cures Everywhere) in Brad's honor, a non-profit organization in Connecticut providing similar sailing opportunities for cancer patients in harbors along Long Island Sound.

I remind you to follow your instincts. Push back. Ask questions. It's your life. You are still in charge.

Complimentary Therapies - At the Cancer Center or Elsewhere

Many cancer centers offer more than just the medical treatment. Unfortunately, they sometimes forget to tell you what's available to you.
- Massage therapy was available to me while having chemo. No need to get undressed. I went with my IV to the massage room. The massage therapist was comfortable and used to dealing with cancer patients. She provided a neck, shoulder, foot massage or reflexology to ease stress.
- Some centers also offer acupuncture, which can help our bodies deal with the side effects of chemo.
- Another complimentary therapy is guided imagery to help your body heal itself.

I also learned that I could come to the center between chemo treatments for hydration when my body needed it. They also offered it to me at home through home health care. This contributed to my feeling much better between treatments because I was not able to get enough food and liquids down. It is even more critical if you are having issues with diarrhea or vomiting.

Scope Out the Minefield -Identify Obstacles

If your job requires you to travel, maybe you have to pass on that for a while. Travel exposes you to very unhealthy environments, such as airports and airplanes. It also chews up a lot of energy. You need all your energy for the healing process.

Lighten up your workload. Don't try to be a martyr and prove to everyone that you can do it. The price is too big to pay. It's false pride. Your goal is to survive. Remember, no one has ever been heard saying on their deathbed. "I wish I had worked more." Most of the regrets are linked to family or self care. Do what you can to remain stimulated without using the energy needed to deal with the treatment and the healing process.

Avoid unhealthy environments and unhealthy people. Remind visitors if they have a cold or are not feeling well, that you should not be exposed to it. Avoid the conference, the meeting, the cocktail party that appeals to you, the trip to Wal-Mart or Target - too many dirty surfaces, too many runny noses, too many germs. If you do have to travel on an airplane, wear a surgical mask to protect yourself and wash your hands the moment you get off the airplane. I make it a practice to wash my hands repeatedly and carry hand sanitizer wherever I go. Other dangerous environments are hospitals and doctor's office. There are a lot of sick people passing through and a lot of germs and viruses. Limit your exposure and keep your hands in your pockets. Watch the contact with hand rails and door knobs.

Surround Yourself with Cheerleaders

Make a list of the people you find uplifting, who believe in you, who admire you. Those who make you laugh. Anyone whose company generally makes you feel better. Call friends for an uplifting session and avoid, at all cost, those who bring you down, who are negative, those whose sympathy is overwhelming when what you want is a piece of normalcy.

CHAPTER 3

HANG IN THERE and BUILD CHARACTER

Cut Yourself Some Slack

You must learn to pamper yourself in many ways.
What brings you pleasure? Make a list.
- A massage
- A soak in the tub
- Fishing
- French pastry or a hot fudge sundae
- Losing yourself in a mystery book
- Going to the movies
- Scrapbooking
- Building something
- An hour at the museum
- Painting
- Writing
- Helping others
- Gardening
- Woodworking

Whatever it is, you may want to add more of these
things in your life.

Acquire an Attitude. Manage Your Thoughts

Know that you can control or reframe your
thoughts. If you don't believe it then ask yourself;
"Who is putting these thoughts in my head?" In
whatever happens in our daily lives, we have the
choice of how we respond to any situation. We can

feel hurt, get upset or we can shrug it off. Other people are not responsible for our behavior and our attitude. We are.

That said, here are some qualities to develop:
Determination: Gain clarity around what you want and keep at it. Stay on course.
Courage: Courage doesn't mean there is no fear. It's the ability to act in the face of fear.
Resilience: The ability to bounce back no matter how far you are stretched. Think of a rubber band. It's the ability to cope with adversity without being destroyed.
Optimism- Some people prefer to look at the down side of things because they don't want to be disappointed. I have found it far more enjoyable to focus on positive outcomes, acting happy, and seeing the glass half full. Focusing on the positives creates hope. Hope makes you feel good and often leads to success.
Spirit: A combination of the above.
Here's a parting thought: Sometimes you can't change the situation, but you can change your attitude towards it. Life is not about waiting for the storm to pass. It's about learning to dance in the rain.

Practice Courage

Why? Because no one likes a whiner (even if you have a good reason).
Because you need to rise above the negative, in order to survive.

You must have a sense of urgency and perspective.
You must believe: I can do it! Keep repeating it
over and over.

Courage reminds me of when I used to downhill ski.
I feared steep hills. I used to stop at the crest of the
hill to work up the courage to go down until I heard
a ski instructor once yell out, "Let's all stand here
and watch the hill get steeper."

That's really what we tend to do. We talk ourselves
out of doing some of the things we know we want
to do because we imagine the worst. We need to
focus on the positive outcomes and identify the little
things we can do, one at a time, to get there.
Courage is not something you acquire which stays
with you like an "aha" moment. It's something you
must work on continuously to maintain.

Take it One Day at a Time

- Find the joy in the moment.
- Wake up every morning and appreciate that
  you are still here.
- If your pain or discomfort is less then
  yesterday, acknowledge it and be grateful.
- Look only at what you have to do today and
  what you would like to do. Think only of
  tomorrow if there is something that you
  must plan to ensure a good day.

- I always enjoyed ABC anchor, Charles Gibson, who closed his World News Report every evening with, "And I hope you had a good day."
- It is a good practice to end every day by taking a few minutes to list the good things that happened today.
- Adopting an "attitude of gratitude" will make you feel better and will help you continue to focus and recognize the good things in your life.
- Savor the moment.
- Don't spend too much time on the big picture.
- I no longer allow the little things to upset me. In the scope of life, they are meaningless.

Be Grateful and Nurture Your Team

Your medical team is critical to your survival. If you think of it, you are vying for their attention with a lot of others. I am always amazed how they remember me, my specific situation and a lot of the little things. I know that my medical oncology team meets with hundreds of patients every week. I want to nurture that relationship so that I stand out in their minds, that they don't mind taking my call, and that they will stretch to help me.

- I bring in cookies, wine, little gifts.
- Tell them that you appreciate their being part of your team.

- Don't cry wolf, otherwise they will hesitate to jump when you are alarmed.
- Respect their time. I was amazed how many times my medical oncologist called me or stopped by the hospital in the evening. He called me several times on a Saturday or Sunday to check up on me or discuss results of a CT scan.

I have never felt, however, that it gave me permission to call his cell phone or   home if I wanted to talk to him. I would call in an emergency.

- I recognize that in oncology they are faced with illness, tragedy, and crisis every day. I want to be the "sunshine" in their day. I work at being upbeat, appreciative, and take the time to dress in colorful, cheerful clothes for an appointment at the cancer center. It works for me.

- I also make a point of going to the websites that rate physicians and facilities and share my positive experience.

- I wrote the president of the institution telling her how impressed and grateful I was with my care providers and listed them by name.

- Take the time to complete and mail in the satisfaction surveys that your cancer center sends out. It is an opportunity for you to give candid feedback. Caregivers and family members can also offer comments on the care received.

- I am a great ambassador for my cancer center and my team.

If You Get Knocked Down – Get Up Again

When my best friend lost her husband to cancer, it was just a few weeks before we were to take a trip to celebrate my 50th birthday. Peter had made me promise to be sure Susan went on the trip if he died beforehand. And so we did. My suggestion to her one morning after a sleepless night, was, "It's ok to cry. You can cry for one hour every day. Then you have to keep busy and occupy yourself."

It's the same with cancer patients. It's OK for us to feel down, to feel whipped, to cry, to feel sad and maybe feel sorry for ourselves – but just for a little while. We've got work to do in order to survive. This is where we apply courage to move forward.

Ask and Accept With Grace

Don't turn people away. If you were offering to help someone in need, how would you feel if you got a quick, "Thanks, but I'm OK"? Trust in your family and friends. Give them a minor assignment. Still better, why not make and maintain a list of what you wish could be done, a list of what you don't feel up to doing yourself. Then when someone offers to help, you can refer to your list and suggest something. Examples might include a ride to the cancer center, picking up ice cream that you wish you had, going to the post office, buying a present

for your mother's birthday. You'll be surprised
how grateful they will be. And you win, too.

I will tell you first hand that this was one of the best
lessons I have learned. I have always prided myself
on being self-sufficient. Feedback from friends is
that they valued my asking for help, sharing my
vulnerability, because their perception is that my
husband and I were always there for them. They
wanted a chance to return the favor.

Emotional Roller Coaster

This is something that both you and those close to
you will experience, and it varies from one person
to another. Some of us react to a crisis by springing
into action rather than focusing on the emotion.
Others need to feel it and deal with it and may
actually be overwhelmed by it, initially or
periodically. Some have developed a great deal of
resilience. Others seem unable to cope with any
adversity.

I found it easier dealing with cancer the first time.
The surprise and the fear made me spring into
action, a natural instinct for me. When I learned that
there was more cancer, a year later, I was so
disappointed. I had just begun to feel comfortable
and safe; that I had beaten it. My husband and I
were both overwhelmed with sadness. We lived
with it, we talked a lot and cried and reached for the
courage to move on. It took me a few weeks to
bounce back to my survivor instincts.

Then, six months later, when my husband tested positive for prostate cancer, I was emotional and depressed. It was one month before my hip replacement surgery, and I was so looking forward to being pain free and getting my life back. I felt that we just couldn't catch a break.

Now that I have experienced a return of cancer, metastases to the brain, pleural drainage, Gamma Knife procedures, serious infection requiring seven months of daily antibiotic infusions, I have become less emotional, more tolerant and generally have less anxiety.
For now, I accept that I am living with cancer (not dying of cancer).

Alternatives to Isolation

Make it a point to get out of the house, even if it's just a ride in the car. Perhaps a friend is running errands and you can enjoy their company and the ride without getting out of the car.

 If you can drive and want to stop at the local drug store, wear a mask if your blood counts are low. Or take advantage of the drug stores that have a drive through. Perhaps you can use the drive through alternative for a mid-morning coffee. Take a walk on your deck or down the street.

Use e-mail to keep in touch with friends and colleagues, share information and experiences. You can chat on the internet with others experiencing the same illness and even gather valuable tips.

Use the telephone to connect with co-workers, colleagues, friends and family. They avoid calling you so as not to disturb you. On the other hand, you are wondering what to do with your time. Give it a try. Most of my friends were delighted to get a call from me.

You can also invite selected visitors. Be sure to caution them not to stop by if they have a cold or virus. Friends and neighbors will probably offer to cook you a meal and deliver it - a good opportunity to socialize.

Grieving is a Natural Reaction

Many of us suffer from grief when facing cancer whether it's the first time around or not. Some of the questions that may run through your mind are:

- Why me?
- Why now?
- What did I do to deserve this?
- How did this happen?
- What is the cause?
- Who is to blame?
- Is this God's way of punishing me?
- How can God allow this to happen to me and my family?

I don't think you will find answers to these questions, nor do I believe you should distract yourself from the challenge at hand. Acknowledge the questions and try to focus on the solutions.

Disappointment is also another emotion. At first it may cause anger and bring on tears. You can give in to it - for a little while. Eventually, you must move on. Do not allow your emotions to paralyze you. I felt a sense of urgency with cancer requiring that I shift into action mode.

A realization that comes as you progress in your journey with cancer is the loss of your personal sense of safety. If you didn't suspect the danger the first time around, how will you know when it returns?

Even when our tumors shrink or dry up, or we are told we are in remission, I believe we are still "living with cancer." Sometimes it will be inactive for a long period, and then it may activate again at any time, with or without warning. I view cancer as a chronic disease, like diabetes or heart condition.

I will forever be cautious going forward, reacting to the smallest change in my body. It is similar to the loss of personal safety that some experience if they have been burglarized, mugged or in a serious car accident. I talk about it with close friends, other cancer patients and I journal about it. I do some self-coaching using techniques I have learned in my career as a coach. Many cancer patients have found counseling from a pastor, a social worker, therapist or support group helpful to move through this grief.

Be Creative

Take a mini-vacation in your mind. Take a few minutes every day, or when you need it most, to imagine yourself at your favorite vacation spot. Play it out. Smell the flowers, the ocean, and the mountains. Pick your favorite restaurant or pastime and feel yourself enjoying that moment. You can either rely on memories or create them yourself.

I enjoy the Caribbean Islands. I love to explore vacation spots on the internet, check lodging and just soak up the beauty of the islands. I maintain a wish list of my favorite spots and decide where I will go when I feel better and have the money. It's like window shopping.

If you have enough concentration to read, get lost in a great novel or good mystery, or watch a movie.

If you have a creative flair, do some scrapbooking, write poetry, knit, crochet, whittle, work on your model trains, learn to juggle or tackle a new craft. Any of this will make you feel productive and will pass the time. I still have hope of learning to juggle.

Pace Yourself- Take a Break

It's OK to cry once in awhile. It's OK to sleep in and take naps. Cut yourself some slack. Stop pushing to live the life you used to. Your energy must be reserved for healing. Don't waste it on work unless your work is stimulating and rewarding. Reinvent yourself; enjoy and cherish the new you.

CHAPTER 4

FACING THE FUTURE

Envision and Design the Future

Plan your 90th birthday party.
Plan your next trip.
Think about the classes you want to take or a new
hobby you want to explore. Even if you can't start
doing it right now, research it.

Count Your Blessings

Make a list.
Observe those around you.
Take the time to smell the roses.
Focus on the glass half full – not half empty.

It's Your Life- You Are Still in Charge

Set boundaries. Get rid of the, "but I have to..." or
"they expect me to..."
Be clear about your personal priorities, your goals.
Is that test or procedure going to help you get there?
If you don't want to have that surgery next week,
reschedule it. Ask yourself whether it is in your
best interest. You have a right to refuse treatment
but do it consciously and knowingly, not with your
head in the sand. Take control of your lifestyle.

Revisit Your Priorities

Your career won't matter if/when you are dead.
Rarely has anyone been heard murmuring on their
deathbed, "I wish I had worked more." So focus:
"Who's on first? What's on second?" What is best
for you, right now? If feeling better, regaining
health is your top priority, then what can you do to
get there?

Make Your Bucket List

If you haven't seen the movie, "The Bucket List,"
with Jack Nicholson, I encourage you to do so. A
bucket list is the list of things you want to do before
you "kick the bucket." What have you always
wanted to do, or you never considered before, but
find it of interest now? Frankly, I think everyone
should have a bucket list, regardless of whether you
are facing your mortality or not.

At one of my visits to my oncologist, I asked what I
should be doing to get back my health, or to prevent
metastasis. His response was, "Do exactly what
you've been doing and have fun." I hear those
words almost daily: Have Fun. Sometimes, just as
I am about to feel guilty about "goofing off" on a
warm sunny beach day, I am reminded that I am
doing exactly what I should be doing, and it's OK.

Acknowledge the Gifts

Since I firmly believe in the importance of a positive outlook when facing challenging odds, it helps to reflect on the good in one's life in order to achieve a balance. Here are the blessings and gifts that I recognize on my journey with cancer.

- Friendships solidified
- Admiration and respect of my peers
- My wonderful supportive husband
- Graciousness and helping hands from neighbors
- Prayers and positive energy from family, friends and colleagues
- Perspective
- Early retirement
- Social Security disability
- Limited discomfort from side effects during chemo
- Surviving a dangerous infection
- My oncology team
- Regaining energy
- Pain-free days
- Patience
- Clinical trials that improved my odds
- Eating chocolate because it feels good

CHAPTER 5

A SPECIAL WORD FOR FAMILY, FRIENDS and CAREGIVERS

So many of you want to help, but you don't know how to begin. What should you say when you hear the news? If you learn about it from the patient, you feel on the spot. You need to respond, and unless you have had the same experience, you simply don't know the right thing to say. It's amazing, isn't it, that even if we have a Master's Degree or a PhD, we probably have never been taught how to deal with sensitive situations or crises.

If you have heard the news through someone else, you have time to prepare your response and reaction. If you are learning the news first hand from the patient, here are some thoughts to keep in mind:

- Call back and acknowledge the situation as soon as possible.
- Sometimes, the patient doesn't want you to say anything. Just listen to them.
- They need to talk it through, in their own time.
- When someone is grieving (and yes we do grieve over the loss of health), we have a need to talk about it, when we are ready, and in an environment where one feels safe.

What You CAN Say:

Did you have any symptoms?
Have you suspected this for a while?
This must be very difficult.
Are you in any pain?
What are you finding the most difficult about your
current situation?
I'm sorry you have to go through this.
Tell me more.
Has it been detected in the early stages?
What is the most frightening part of this for you?
Is this something you want to share with others – or
is it confidential?
What do you find most overwhelming that you
could use help with?
Is it OK if I check in with you regularly to see how
you are doing and how I can help?
You have a great attitude (or stamina, or courage). I
am sure this will help you.
Your attitude and courage are an inspiration.
I would like to make and bring you over a few
meals for those days that you don't feel like
cooking, is that ok?
I am available to drive you to a doctor's
appointment or pick up a prescription for you. Call
me at any time.
Is there someone you would like me to call for you?
What type of chores around the house could you use
some help with?

What NOT to Say:

I'm sure you'll get through it without a problem.
It could be worse. I know a friend that...
Thank God it's not ...
What you should do immediately is...
You should call my doctor.
I don't know what I would do if it happened to me.
I think I would rather die.
Oh my God -you must be devastated.
I would never consider chemo – I would try only
natural remedies.
I heard that if you eat asparagus every day it will
cure your cancer.

Don't play it down. Don't compare it to others,
except from an informative, educational
perspective. In the beginning, avoid telling us about
someone else we know who had this and died.
We're not ready for that kind of news.

What You Can Do:

- Be present for us, even if only to listen. We don't expect you to rescue us. And don't be uncomfortable if we cry. Lend us your shoulder. Lend us your ear. Give us a hug. Give us hope.

- If the person wants to share information with family and friends, you could set up a blog on Caringbridge.org. Why? To limit the number of people calling the house and the burden of returning calls to well-meaning people.

- If you know others who have experienced similar cancer and/or treatment, connect them. That cancer survivor is usually much more informed than you are on the topic.

- Cook healthy, easy-to-eat meals that can be frozen or easily reheated.
    - Focus on comfort food: soups, stews and casseroles are great choices.
    - Meals can be packaged in serving sizes rather than a large quantity to feed 8, unless of course they have a large family.
    - Ask about food restrictions or preferences.
    - Cookies are great to nibble on, or share with visitors.
    - You probably don't want to send a fruit basket or flowers to a cancer patient in treatment. Why? Because after chemo their

blood count might drop and they may have to avoid raw fruit and vegetables.

- When I was having radiation, I was told to use skin care products that do not contain metals. Most cosmetics do. If you can find body lotion, shower gel or shampoos at the natural health store, that would be a nice gift. Be sure to verify that it contains no metal.

- Funny movies on video might be appreciated.

- Audio books might be easier than reading, because of concentration levels.

- Help the caregivers, too. I have often felt that it might be more difficult being the caregiver than the patient. The patient's attention is focused on this overwhelming activity in their life. The caregiver supports and observes, but cannot change the situation, and that is very difficult. You can offer to be at the house so they can feel comfortable going out. There may be a need to have someone available in case of a problem, even if the patient is sleeping. Or perhaps, it's just about making the caregiver comfortable. Even if the patient does not need company, the caregiver may need company and support.

- Offer to do chores. Even if they decline initially, offer again later. Most people automatically decline help and rarely ask. A cancer patient has to learn to accept help and it might take a while. Here are a few chores that could help:

> Cutting the lawn, pruning the shrubs, planting some flowers.
> Vacuuming, washing the kitchen and bathroom floors.
> Washing the windows.
> Taking out the trash.
> Doing the laundry.

Maybe they would be uncomfortable with you doing this work. Perhaps you will need to assure them you have the time to do this and you would like to see them save their energy for healing.

Another option might be to send your own housecleaner over as a gift or give them a gift certificate for housecleaning. There's an organization called "Cleaning for a Reason" where patients can get a free housecleaning while in treatment. (cleaningforareason.org)

When I lost a great deal of weight, I asked for hand-me-down clothes from anyone who might have outgrown their clothes. I needed sizes 6 and 8 temporarily. Two people obtained clothes from a friend and offered them to me. One friend bought and sent me two velour pant suits with coordinated turtle neck sweaters. These were ideal for chemo days or just for lounging at home. Sometimes you just have to take action – without asking.

- Buy an uplifting audio book about cancer, hope, complimentary therapies, and nutrition for cancer patients.
- Give a gift certificate for complimentary massage, reflexology or facial. Make it close to their home or at the cancer center.

You simply cannot know how valuable your support is. The ongoing encouragement, positive thoughts, e-mails, cards, little gifts and remembrances are the fuel that keeps us going. Your caring attitude, your friendship, and your prayers are welcome and greatly appreciated.

Caring for the Caregiver

The following are excerpts from an article by Jai Pausch, in "Cancer Today", a patient advocate, primary caregiver for her late husband, Randy, who authored the acclaimed, "The Last Lecture" following his diagnosis with pancreatic cancer.

Beyond the support of family and friends, where can a new caregiver turn for guidance? In our case, Randy's oncologist recommended a counselor, who helped me create successful strategies for addressing the emotional challenges we faced during treatment, remission, recurrence and death.

I also learned that finding another caregiver of similar life circumstances can ease the sense of isolation many caregivers experience. My brother introduced me to a woman with two young children whose husband had a rare cancer that had metastasized to his liver. She understood exactly what I was going through: fear of widowhood and single parenthood, juggling of domestic responsibilities with medical care, confusion over treatments and side effects and uncertainty about the future.

I could never have made it through 23 months as a caregiver if it had not been for the many kinds of help I received. As you face this same journey, remember: There are many helpful hands waiting to reach out and support you.

You can help the caregiver by suggesting a list of tasks you can and want to do. Perhaps you can pick up groceries. Take the kids to soccer practice. Organize a meal webpage (try foodtidings.com). Help out with laundry. Don't just say: "Call me if you need anything."

Offer a distraction, like a ball game or a movie, with no cancer talk. Help the caregiver take a break and feel like a normal person.

About the Author

Margot Larson is a personal and professional coach, helping people face challenges in their careers, and business leaders dealing with workplace issues. The author has already done due diligence in facing her own illness, Stage 4 inoperable and recurrent Lung Cancer along with side effects impacting her career and mobility. Margot is proud to be counted among the five year survivors.

The author is known by her friends and peer group as a coach who can turn chaos into acceptable "bites", who can bring hope, ideas and direction to most situations. She has been an inspiration to her personal and business network, as seen in testimonials on her www.caringbridge.org site.

Margot authored *"Jump Start Your Life"*, about choosing your own lifestyle before someone chooses it for you.

53240357R00043

Made in the USA
San Bernardino, CA
10 September 2017